THE D

SEX
THE DONE THING

Drusilla Beyfus
Cartoons by Austin

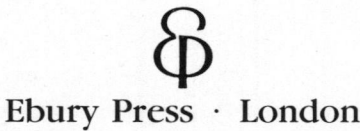

Ebury Press · London

First published 1993

1 3 5 7 9 10 8 6 4 2

Text copyright © Drusilla Beyfus 1993
Illustrations copyright © David Austin 1993
Drusilla Beyfus has asserted her right under the Copyright,
Designs and Patents Act, 1988, to be identified as the author of
this work.

All rights reserved. No part of this publication may be
reproduced, stored in a retrieval system, or transmitted in any
form or by any means, electronic, mechanical, photocopying,
recording or otherwise, without prior permission of the
copyright owners.

First published in the United Kingdom in 1993 by
Ebury Press Limited
Random House, 20 Vauxhall Bridge Road, London SW1V 2SA

Random House Australia (Pty) Limited
20 Alfred Street, Milsons Point, Sydney,
New South Wales 2061, Australia

Random House New Zealand Limited
18 Poland Road, Glenfield
Auckland 10, New Zealand

Random House South Africa (Pty) Limited
PO Box 337, Bergvlei, South Africa

Random House UK Limited Reg. No 954009

A CIP catalogue record for this book
is available from the British Library

ISBN 0 09 178237 6

Filmset by SX Composing Ltd, Rayleigh, Essex

Printed in by England by Clays Ltd, St Ives plc

To M., with love

Contents

Preface 1   Eros's try 2

Her move 5   Love nest 6

Mementos 8   Wow! 10

Food of love 13   First time 16

Safe-ish sex 19   Whistling man 22

Minority report 24   Dating game 27

Peacockry 30   Meet the folks 31

Toy boy 34   Unavailable 35

Kiss 'n' sell 38   Bedroom bliss 40

Two is company 41   Betrayal 43

Afterthought 46   'Bye 48

No go 49

Preface

Etiquette and sex, on the surface, are strange bedfellows. One is cool, the other hot. The former is about restraint, the latter about release. Convention prompts the first which gives way to physical urges and biology.

Nevertheless, collaboration between the two has always been fruitful. Good manners, in any case, do have a bearing on love-making. Tact, understanding and reassurance are as much parts of a lover's prerogatives as the unbridled passions.

Few doubt that the ground rules of the mating game are in disarray. Many claim they don't know how to make new acquaintances or how to proceed when boy meets girl. Belle has become Beau in many respects, showing a penchant for making the running in ways that are thought masculine. Yet, by the same token, women show little enthusiasm for being considered forward. Men may find that the Old Adamistic approach raises eyebrows and nothing else, which means a rethinking of strategies.

Manners are in the making in many fields. The social mingling of gaydom with the world of straights in a more open way is but one example. Another concerns the preliminaries involved in embarking on a sexual relationship with a new partner. Sensitive questions have to be put to the other, touched off by concern about HIV and STDs.

As part of this precautionary approach, women have

had to learn to look after their welfare in a more practical manner and turn condom-bearer. Some finesse is required if an emotional spark is not to be quenched by clinical considerations.

Cupid is having his work cut out these days. There are so many points of difference between people that put the other beyond the pale. An amorous prospect may die the death through an unconsidered remark, now that Political Correctness places such an inhibiting brake on conversation. A *tendresse* for the other could bite the dust over a divergence of food attitudes. Then again, romantic yearnings are liable to go up in smoke when the beloved flouts the other's no-smoking caveats. Bridges will have to be built or people will have to be satisfied with an extremely short list of possible mates.

Underlying the recommendations on these pages is the fond hope that good manners enable lovers to feel more comfortable with one another. This seems a good start for getting as close as can be.

Eros's try

Making the first moves in a relationship is always razor-edged. The risk of cutting rejection has to be balanced against gut impulse. No guarantees of success will be proffered below but some approaches would seem to stand a better chance than others.

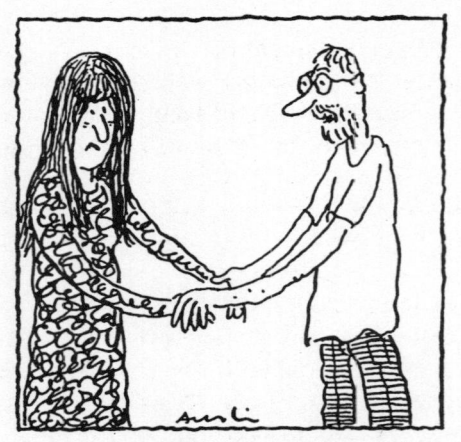

Have you got another significant other?

Part of the dilemma is that many of the old ground rules in the mating game have been lost or abandoned. One example might be at a club dance. Time was when it would be quite acceptable for a partner to ask a woman that he fancied and whom he didn't know, for a turn on the dance floor. Many doubts might choke back such a request nowadays, or others in a similar vein. Will he be thought forward, naff, sexist or overkeen? Yet his fancied partner may well be longing to be asked for a number.

Approaches are invariably easier on the basis of shared friends or acquaintances or colleagues. It might be possible for a shy partner to introduce himself as a friend of X or Y.

Chat-up techniques based on the more obvious manifestations of the Old Adam may suit some but they carry the stigma of insensitivity, and lack of imagination. Any opening line of conversation is more promising, on the face of it, than one that remarks on a woman's bosom, legs or derrière. What is wanted is an approach that flatters the listener's levels of thought.

Asking someone for a drink is a time-honoured pick-up ploy, but has the disadvantage that once refused, there is nowhere to go. In a group, once again, the services of a third party can be invaluable. A pal of the smitten can dispatch a message via an intermediary – and no face is lost if the offer is declined.

'Looks' between two, the standby of romantic novelists, can leap amazing distances, cut a swathe through crowds and may command attention in a trice. A negative from the recipient can be expressed in the bat of an eyelid or an uninterested returning gaze, all without a word having to be spoken. A smile that accompanied an accepting response would be most encouraging.

In an age of studied casualness, males may be reminded that women like to be the subject of special attentions. Formal means of declaring an interest would be to send flowers, write a letter, issue invitations, and of course telephone. It is doubtful if tangible presents are acceptable between virtual strangers, but exceptions might include snapshots of the party, or any personal token of the occasion/event/study course which brought you two together.

Her move

It may be argued that women have gained a great deal of leeway in overtly making the pace in a love affair. That said, uncertainties do exist as far as making initial advances are concerned. She may and does propose a first date but the manner of the approach matters.

Well within limits surely is that a female may make the telephone call that follows up a first meeting. If she wants to propose a date there are circumspect suggestions and those that might seem to overstep the mark. Acceptable is to suggest going out together with friends, making up a party, asking him home for a meal or a drink at which others will be present, mentioning you will look out for him at the disco. More equivocal invitations because the emphasis is on your presence rather than the occasion might be to propose a solo invitation, or yourself as a date for a party. Dropping in at his place uninvited takes a very cool head and one that dares a rebuff.

Not every woman favours a diplomatic approach to dating. A breed of female is making itself known that prefers an upfront, right on, and no-nonsense-about-flirtation style. It may be guessed that the male has reservations about Jill, the lad. But the approach wins

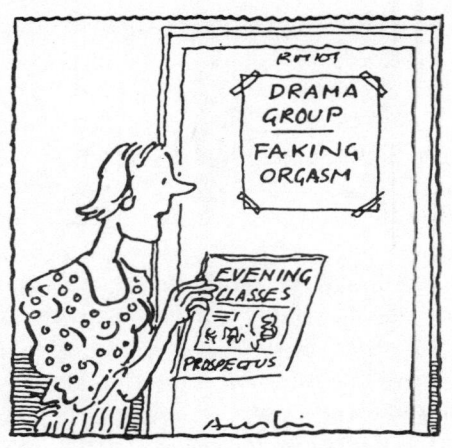

some, from all accounts. One factor has to be borne in mind by free spirits. If she wants to make it like one of the boys she should be prepared to take any flak like a man.

Love nest

No doubt passion can hold its own upon a mossy bank, beside the lapping shores or aboard a punt. That being said, no one should underestimate the value of preparing a love nest.

Those who invite the object of their affections to stay

over at home are advised to put some thought into making the place worthy of its status as a Temple of Love.

Privacy should be inviolate. Ensure that the promise of a time together alone is exactly that. Likely droppers-in should be strongly discouraged in advance. No visits from Mum, best girlfriend/ally, nosy neighbour, siblings should be entertained. An acceptable excuse for not asking in a caller is domestic chaos – people flee at the prospect of being asked to help. In general, the less said the better. Other standbys include an impending hot telephone call from the boss; attending to your wretched tax affairs; just wanting to be alone for a while; or saying simply you can't talk now.

Regretfully, the house canine may have to be parked with a friend who owes you one. A call for gumboots and a long walk in the rain in order to water Rover may come later but isn't on the bill tonight.

The telephone can be doused in cushions, the fax disconnected, but the answerphone may do good service with the proviso that the volume for incoming calls is turned down.

Television can represent serious competition in amorous adventures. Recommended: the programme listings are studied circumspectly in advance. If the chosen date of the rendezvous coincides with a big match or fight, a female may have her work cut out to remain No 1. Similarly, the culmination of a drama series or favourite soap may well take priority over other diversions for her.

Videos, however, as their timing is at the behest of the viewer, may agreeably lengthen waking hours, be they blue, monotone or straight colour.

The bed itself, it goes without saying, should be temptingly fresh, soft and welcoming, ideally endowed with a sultanesque profusion of pillows.

Conspicuous evidence of a recent amorous attachment is best removed. Left-behind tights/underpants, hairpins/shaving tackle in the bathroom, remains of old bottles of scent/aftershave — OUT. Similarly, any snapshots of the ex-favourite might seem spare, particularly if the affair was recent.

The aim is to create surroundings in an attempt to do justice to the moment in which present company comes first.

Mementos

Presents for the desired one require taste, timing and imagination. Effective offerings should be a glorious surprise. Whatever the cash value of the gesture, it should exude an unstinting wish to please.

As far as timing is concerned, a golden rule is the sooner the better. The offering may enhance the prospects of the giver. Evidence of an ability to discern the G-spot of preference is a great point in favour. In some

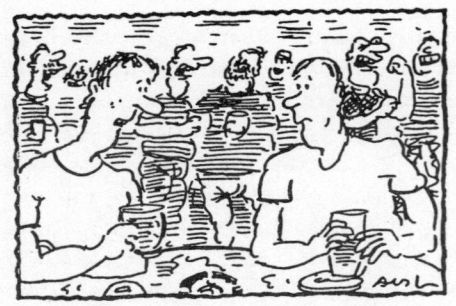

I scored – but not very high, it seems.

cases, like-mindedness in the field of style and taste has a dynamic comparable to sexual compatability.

The many givers who might be down on their financial luck but who are in a giving mood are advised to major on forethought and effort. Hunting down a nice little something that doesn't cost will of its nature show determination not to be defeated by being short of the readies. Also, detail with perky paper and ribbons and card can be attended to, but a word of warning here – an exuberantly wrapped box of biscuits may be thought a distinct downer.

Some suggestions with appeal for either sex: a hat, the first of the season's white lilac, sweet peas or narcissi; a wished-for copy of a sought-after out-of-print book; initialled cufflinks or tie-pin; a cornucopia of standby supplies from a reliable deli; CDs or cassettes of music to taste; an unusual but house-trained plant; a collection of paperbacks by a favourite author; a video of a lamented missed television programme; a flashy umbrella; a T-shirt with core logo; exotic soap; decorative candlesticks; beeswax candles; approved bottled smells; a dress ring for sentiment's sake; a limited edition print by an admired painter or photographer; a photo album filled with snaps of the darling one; a chic collar for the house canine or moggy; good seats for a coveted show; a recipe excellently hand-made by the giver for a grand nosh-up.

On the other hand, the offer to repair the windscreen, bang up some shelving, fix the refrigerator or rewire the desk lamp might have fantastic sex appeal.

Wow!

Sexy dress for females is as interesting as ever despite — or perhaps because of — the genderless air that has descended on apparel in general.

Played right, overtly seductive attire can help to transform a plain body, but give it an inch and you are in the realm of sleaze.

The whole question of sexuality in dress is complex, much residing in the eye of the beholder. On one level the subject shades into the darker side of fetishism and deviance, on another, into the acceptable attractions of everyday black tights.

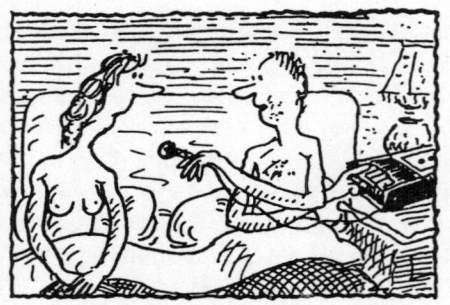

Just for the record – how was it for you?

Two factors are likely to shape success. Guessing the predilection of the loved one accurately and relating whatever is to be worn to the time and the place.

No one can predict such a personal area of choice on behalf of another. But if a suspicion is entertained that the dress/outfit/skirt/top is likely to raise eyebrows in an uncomplimentary fashion, try it out on a reliable ally before putting hopes to the test. In general, dress is more seductive than undress and by the same token, a hint has greater powers of allure than total revelation. At a time when legs, thighs, backs, bosoms and midriffs are parts of the body which fashion legitimately exposes, a prudish approach has little to recommend it. However, a sense of discrimination about the options is the order of the day, usually endorsed by the boys. At least as far as their own beloved is concerned. A visible panty line has few admirers, by the way.

An important consideration is the mixed-up plural nature of fashion and social life. A sassy outfit that might well have its moments in a Soho disco may strike an unseemly note at the subscription or club dance. Club members, as a rule, might find it hard to see the joke.

Formality on the whole still spells a cautious approach to risqué attire. Formal dos, receptions, office parties, business entertaining, meeting friends of the beloved when it is specially important to create a good impression, are doubtful occasions.

Discos, private parties and dances and informal get-togethers are opportunities to test the waters of acceptability. Appropriateness is always a trusted guide but this can lead to cloned dress. Self-expression shouldn't be forgotten as an indicator of personality.

If the maximum impact is to be gained from a red hot dress, self-confidence is all. Nervous attempts to modify the wow factor will only serve to draw attention to the wearer's doubts about her choice.

The last word has to be that it is the wearer who breathes allure into inanimate apparel. Some people – it is one of the unfairnesses of life – possess that perceived quality even when they put on any old thing.

Food of love

An invitation to eat at home has long signalled a wish on the part of the inviter to know his or her guest better. If the occasion is to be dinner for two, or perhaps lunch, the stage is set for cooking up a romance.

Fanning a friendship without seeming blatant about intentions is always a delicate matter. Asking someone to dinner is a handy card as the invitation has a far more intimate air than meeting in a public spot, and offers the host a chance to show his or her colours.

With a reputation as a friend, a host, a cook and provider at stake, the occasion is one that takes some forethought if all is to go as wished. Certainly, it would seem very uncool to betray any undue concern during the occasion about the success of the outcome. The ideal is for things to seem unfussed and natural.

A few caveats to begin with. Skip the idea of asking the guest in advance what they would like to eat and drink. The chances are it will present difficulties to the interrogated to guess what is within the scope of their friend's resources, the depth of his or her pocket and the inviter's ideas of hospitality. No, this is an occasion for the party giver to lead the way firmly and decide what is fit. An exception might be double-checking on whether the guest is a veggie or a carnivore. In either case, the recommendation is to go with the friend's preference, as apart from

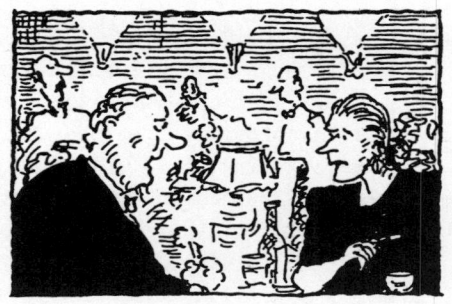

Don't you think food is the finest foreplay?

anything else there doesn't seem much point in starting off under the shadow of a divisive topic.

It might also be circumspect to give foods a miss on this occasion that are known to present an etiquette puzzle as to the proper way to go about eating them. Likewise, to give a wide berth to dishes liable to create whiffy breath, buttery chins or spinachy smiles.

Culinary ideas will come from outside these pages, but it is worth thinking about whether conventional advice is sound. Choosing a humdrum, tried-and-tested approach may simplify the cook's role but it discounts the dangers of an untimely snap between a boring menu and the mind of the host. A more interesting dish than those in one's usual repertoire – assuming a limited range – might speak volumes.

A compromise is to go for one course that takes careful timing or last-minute titivation, for example, and to aim to keep the rest of the meal dead simple. A glorious pud is always an attraction, looks pretty and shows effort.

One of the unsung advantages of playing cook is that ready excuses exist for nipping out to keep an eye on the cooking — any awkward silences can be broken diplomatically in this way. Nevertheless, solo diners do grow restive if the cook vanishes for long without explanation.

On the question of guestly offers to help: probably best declined as a rule as in no time at all proceedings can descend to canteen level.

What to serve to drink is obviously an important consideration. Overdoing the amount is a temptation when much may be at stake, but easy does it. A heavy hand on the pouring could mean an unfortunate end to aspirations. A knowledgeable choice of bottle of wine is likely to be appreciated by the man or woman who knows (or who would like to be thought of as knowing) their regional makes and vintages. A glass of something specially good at the end of the meal when the host is feeling more relaxed, comes at the right moment.

If the effort that has gone into satisfying the inner man or woman is to be done justice to, the other arrangements will probably need attention. The classic standbys of candlelight, fresh flowers and music (ensure that this last is keenly attuned to the visiting ear) will all help to heighten a sense of occasion.

No mention so far of aphrodisiacs as an ingredient for an amorous exercise. There is a strong case for thinking that if a pinch of powdered rhino horn or crushed beetle shard in the menu is compulsive, then the gods were against the affair.

As far as our guest is concerned, he or she should arrive punctually, bringing a bottle if wished. Good guests express appreciation in the here and now, show no inclination to truculence, offer to help but gracefully desist if the gesture is declined, and aim to give the impression they can't wait to see more of you.

First time

The psychological stage when a couple have first made love is often a twilit land. Neither may have any clear idea of the other's intentions, nor where it all might be leading.

Assuming that the man is footloose and fancy free (extra-curricular liaisons put a different perspective on proceedings), how best may he judge the borderlines between making assumptions and appearing wimpish?

Feminine psychology may be variable, but few women do not appreciate being appreciated. Among endearing approaches would be a telephone call as soon as possible after parting, and certainly not later than the day after. Hearts will go out to a suitor who manages to overcome all the glitches that proverbially attend those who want to get through to someone urgently.

Flowers are a good idea as a rule but senders should ensure that if the bouquet is to be delivered to a home address, someone will be available to take it in. In the likely event of no one being at home, it would be better to send to the workplace, all depending. A bonus here is that the bunch may help to stir a little mystery into the day's routine, at least as far as curious witnesses are concerned.

A note handwritten by the giver is a more heart-warming memento than either a pre-printed card or one that is dictated to the florist. Besides, some self-conscious donors may hesitate to express themselves as lovingly as they might have done, had they been the writer.

This introduces the topic of the need for diplomacy in public utterance at this point. Most people like to keep new moves in their love lives to themselves for a while. It would certainly be bad manners to spread the word without consulting the other person in the case. We are only thinking of a liaison that is likely to last a while, as the idea of broadcasting casual conquests is surely boys' own stuff.

One word about using office communications technology for very private messages. The answerphone may be hazardous as breathy missives recorded between business-ese have a habit of sounding comically inappropriate when played back in the matter-of-fact environment of the workplace. A similar source of

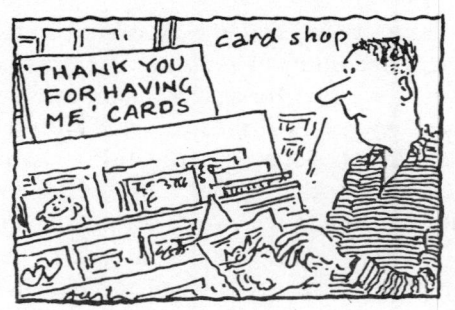

embarrassment is the beloved who fancies the idea of leaving an intimate message on the misguided assumption that the recipient will pick his or her moment to listen in. But it is a fact of office life that answerphones are often used with the sound permanently turned up to full volume; not a kiss will be missed! In cases where this happens at some formal meeting, the only response of the recipient is to treat the matter lightheartedly at the moment and to offer tacit apologies.

The fax machine likewise churns out stuff for general consumption as well as communications addressed to individuals, and often the two get mixed or mislaid, or more likely than not left lying about for anyone to read. However, car phones are a lover's boon as the conversation is likely to be private – at least at the driver's end.

On another tack, presents to commemorate the occasion seem to belong to another more gracious era, but no harm in following the idea. For women, jewellery has a long history of marking seduction. But in this case as in others it might seem to be making assumptions. The recipient, also, might feel that acceptance of the present might be misinterpreted as indicating a commitment that was far from her mind.

When all is said and done, what women want to hear is that they are simply delicious and infinitely interesting, both in mind and body. The important part is for such endearing sentiments to be shared and not kept for private reflection only.

Verbal communication has its limits though, especially on the occasion of making it with a new partner for the first time. It seems doubtful if it is a good idea to interrogate him or her on whether they enjoy this, that or the other form of love-making. It might be more rewarding to trust to instinct and talk later.

Safe-ish sex

It may be some compensation to know that sex was never safe, as the tale of the Garden of Eden testifies. All that has happened is that we are infinitely more aware of the need to protect ourselves from the negative consequences of carnal embrace. What is on offer to this end may be described as safe-ish sex, the best we can do by way of damage limitation.

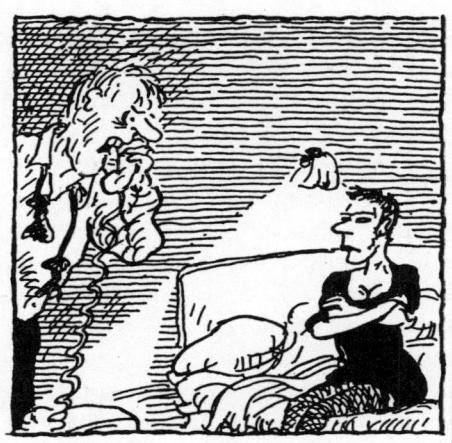

*It is an emergency, doctor.
She insists on a blood test.*

What has to be managed by ordinary mortals is the supremely sensitive task of combining a love of romance with the requirements of 'safe' sex. For the shadows of AIDS, the HIV virus as well as other STDs (sexually transmitted diseases), not to mention unwanted pregnancy, have fallen over the encounter from the first fine careless rapture. Preliminaries in love-making have rarely called for greater tact and discrimination. Questions about a partner's sexual bill of health and the availability of condoms or barriers have become lovers' conversation. The interrogation is at its most delicate when a couple contemplate their first-time together experience, a consideration in its own right. One lighthearted recommendation from a trier is to seal the lips with a kiss and pop a hard question, kiss and repeat. The idea is right if the methodology highly personal.

It is said that women in particular hold back from venturing the practical enquiries. The grounds are that this might be intrusive or seem to presume upon an intimacy that did not exist in the mind of the other, thereby spoiling an atmosphere of trust. In the case of a serious fancy being involved, the ability to judge the timing of what is premature and what is belated is of the essence.

Partners should surely keep their protectives close by the field of engagement. Having to forage in a remote handbag, disappear into the bathroom or search for a wallet is not what the poets had in mind.

Women who are going out with a favourite are usually able to divine the way the wind is blowing. They are advised in these circumstances to carry condoms, just in case. No need to blazon the fact in advance, however.

Another eventuality that needs considering is when one of the partners has an infection or has symptoms that suggest he or she may have caught an STD from the other. It is worse than discourteous to stay mum on the matter. When either or both of a couple are troubled in this way, mutual reassurance is in order, and acceptance that abstinence is a precaution until a medic's all-clear is sounded.

What makes many of the potentially sensitive themes

less so is the widespread generality of the human dilemma in an age in which health awareness is equalled by a free-for-all appetite for sex. All the human problems are dissected, recognised, talked about and written about exhaustively, and to this extent, any public embarrassment surrounding condom culture has had its day. The private individual, however, has to find his or her own way through the libidinous maze.

Whistling man

Since the first human wolf walked, man has whistled at female pulchritude. Whereas in polite circles at least, the call has never been considered anything but laddish — oafish even — whistlers move in a changed climate nowadays. If the male goes too far, misjudges his subject, or timing, he risks giving offence. In certain cases, his job may be on the line or he may provoke an official rebuke, as a recent controversial court case underlined.

What has changed the public mood is woman's objection to such braggadocio responses to their womanly physique. What ires them is the male assumption that such attentions will be welcome, focusing as these do on what is seen as a crude view of their sex.

Nevertheless, defenders claim that the gesture is virtually harmless, and is merely a virile response of the male to the attractions of the opposite sex. In favour also

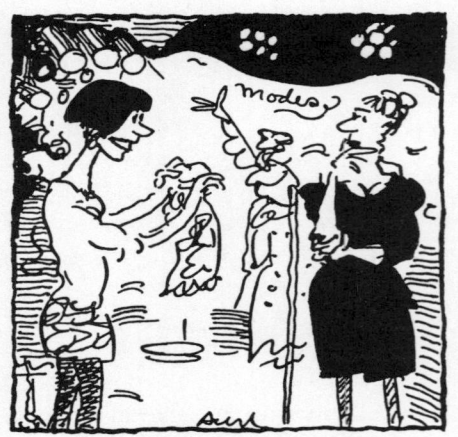

I'd like to try it on and walk past a building site in it.

is that not all women feel so strongly about the matter. Some publicly admit to feeling quite flattered by the attention.

Establishing limits is difficult because much depends on the context. In general, women have fair grounds for raising objections when as the result of attracting lewd whistles they appear to lose dignity or professional clout.

As a rule, women are unaccompanied by men when whistlers do their thing, but should this not be the case, the escort can glare meaningfully at the teaser. Women are advised to keep their eyes straight ahead and to ignore the blandishment.

On the other hand, if the mood inclines, a smile may be in order.

Minority report

Gays are mingling with others in a much more open manner, calling for a social code that takes note of the fact. The absence of secrecy about homosexuality, however, by no means dispenses with the uses of discretion all round.

It is not on to ask a person if they are gay or have 'come out'. A general rule of courtesy, notwithstanding the author's present comments, is to avoid singling out people on grounds of their sexual orientation. Arch proponents of gay pride will disagree.

Loaded remarks about queens, queers or poofters are liable to offend straights as well as those to whom the tag is intended to refer. Of course, humans will always say what they think in terms that they know best despite the onrush of political correctness in these matters. A guideline is to judge the audience well, remembering that circumstances, as usual, alter cases. What would be considered crass are remarks that showed an unawareness of any personal sensitivities involved.

Similarly, it would be discourteous and could be damaging to disclose publicly any private knowledge of a person's homosexual leanings. A reservation to be

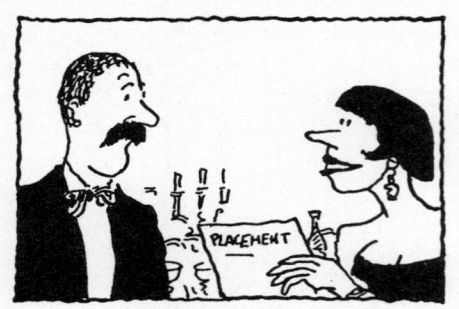

*Would you prefer to be
a boy or a girl at dinner?*

observed rigorously at the workplace and among the person's family.

Approaches differ between parents of self-declared gays on the matter of going public. In instances in which the offspring has come out, parents have no need to make the point. Others may broach the matter obliquely and mention that their son 'moves in gay circles', leaving others to draw their own conclusions.

Gay couples need considering in relation to the party scene, structured as this is on heterosexual codes. Courtesy is to invite a gay guest and his named friend if both are known to the inviter. At a formal dinner party with equal numbers, the party-giver might ask her gay invitee to bring a woman friend, or might fill the gap from the guest list. Or, as is increasingly the habit, the host might accept odd numbers of guests.

On the occasion of a gay couple being invited to stay, it would be thoughtful to ask them if they would like to share, or occupy separate bedrooms. Space permitting, of course. It could be mistaken to make assumptions. However, should members be present who might be discomfited by conspicuous sharing arrangements, separation would seem the right decision. A cover is that it is customary for persons of the same sex to bunk down together for a short stay, with no special inferences drawn. This seems the place to note that not everyone takes a liberal view of gaydom. Gay lovers are expected to abide by the code that governs the others, which is of going easy on public gestures of affection in situations where members stand to be embarrassed.

An aspect of homosexual coupledom as yet unconsidered is the tragic incidence of AIDS among the gay community. Outsiders may wonder whether it is acceptable to ask if someone suffers from the HIV virus. A guideline is to wait to be told. In a letter of condolence to friends and family of an AIDS fatality it would probably be best to omit any reference to the cause of death. The letter to someone who has lost a lover and helpmeet should reflect those very considerations.

Much of the above advice applies in spirit if not according to specifics, to lesbian friends.

Dating game

Of all blind dates the one between two who have signed up with a dating agency carries the greatest investment of hope and risk.

Finding a partner through a professional introduction requires a measure of self-honesty that does not always come naturally in emotional affairs. Recommendations are to state candidly your likes and dislikes as far as a prospective partner is concerned. Questions to be answered in the paperwork may concern political leanings (more left-wing women than men are on the books), education and background. One agency goes so far as to check on preferred alcoholic drinks.

Smokers face a hard time, here as everywhere. It is probably wiser for a declared lover of the weed to indicate a preparedness to try to abstain. Even chain smokers are said to shun those who share their foible.

Another luckless group is women over forty-five. Sadly, many agencies will not allow them on the books as experience suggests they have little chance of being chosen. However, it seems unreasonable to assume that all women in this category are the same; interested parties take note. If an attempt at deception is contemplated the chances of being rumbled should be a prior consideration. The caveat does not apply to men who are formally granted a longer spell of desirability.

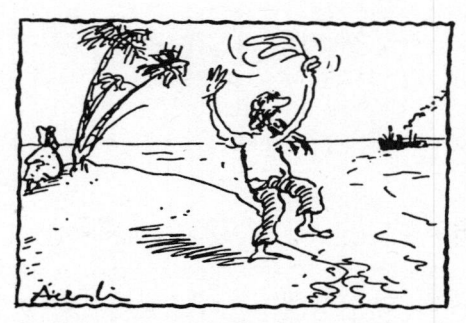

Thank heavens – somebody to introduce us.

As the majority of introductions are largely sparked by the photograph of the client supplied, it makes sense to produce a good likeness. One leading agency described the ideal impression as 'happy and natural'. Enhanced reality is the aim here; giving a totally false impression is liable to rebound to the subject's embarrassment.

Once a partner has been chosen, procedures follow those of any other social engagement. Telephone calls are exchanged (to be made at sociable hours only) and letters written (to be answered as a matter of courtesy). If preliminaries go well, either side can suggest a meeting. Neutral ground is best, such as foregathering at a pub, wine bar or café, or going for a stroll in the park. Invitations to the other's abode at this early stage is thought unwise.

Topics of conversation should have an emphasis on the light and friendly and be respectful. Tales of loss, redundancy and marital break-up are probably best swallowed. On the other hand, some genuine feeling and background information must seep through if only as a basis upon which to decide to take matters a stage further.

In the instance of a date being a flop, courtesy is to stay around for the agreed time. A previously established hour of departure is crucial as protection against uncongenial company and boredom. As far as paying for any hospitality is concerned, going dutch is usual. But in the event of one party graciously offering to pick up the bill – so be it.

Opting out is known to be the catch. Difficult indeed. Polite put-offs are to call it a day with some remark such as 'I'll call sometime'. Those with more courage and the kinder cut might thank the person for his or her company, mention that it has been good to talk but that they don't see a continuing relationship as a possibility. People do understand, but any rejection should be put in the nicest way.

As to a quick sexual fling, it is interesting that even the agencies counsel against. For one thing the pros do not accept responsibility for any untoward outcome as the result of these introductions. Very careful screening is an obvious precaution on both sides.

Peacockry

The time may not be far off when men may ask to borrow their fancy's make-up bag for a quick refresher. And no eye-brows raised. Indeed, as with women, it will be taken as a sign of wishing to keep up appearances in the company of the beloved.

As at present the latest manifestation of male peacockry is confined to the rock, pop, style and fashion milieus, manners are very much in the making as far as a wider audience is concerned. Likely guidelines can be found in society's attitude to women who advanced the cause of cosmetics earlier in this century. As late as the Twenties, it must be said, commentators found amusement in the spectacle of a bright young thing coolly powdering her nose before the impassive gaze of her escort, in a smart restaurant.

As a form of mating display, the old rules will probably apply. Few embargos exist about what can be carried off with aplomb in private, or at a private gathering in the company of those who feel comfortable with the practice. In public, there will always be critics who associate men who take grooming to such an extent with the taint of effeminacy, and on this score the practice runs the risk of being a turn-off.

One caveat in cases of cheating: lipstick marks on a collar, an unfamiliar perfume on night clothes, rouge on

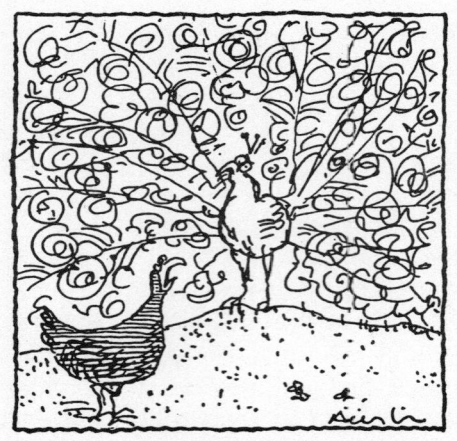

I'd prefer something similar, but in brown.

a kerchief, all long-considered tell-tale signs of man's infidelity, may become subject to gender-bending and apply to either sex.

Meet the folks

Recommended for lovers on meeting the parents of the loved one for the first time: steer by the rules of courtship even if the word does not apply in a conventional sense. Whether the boyfriend or girlfriend in question is contemplating matrimony or an affair, parents are likely to feel protectively towards their offspring, whatever age she or he may be.

A few ground rules apply. It would be courteous if the newcomer gave the impression at least that he or she had been looking forward to the meeting. If goodwill is sought, showing tender concern for the object of his or her desire can only go down well. It is also suggested that the visitor should show a sense of caring about what sort of figure he or she cuts in the eyes of the parents. This last not just for his or her own sake, but out of respect for the loved one's wish for warm approval to be given.

An attempt to find out the interests or predilections of the parents in advance would be friendly and provide some common ground for chat beyond the topic of the loved one. It is an occasion to tread warily over known controversial issues but not to retreat into wimpishness or wetness for the sake of politesse, which probably wouldn't wash anyway.

If the first invitation is for a meal at home it might be an idea to bring a bottle or flowers. Arrive punctually and don't leave conspicuously early without a convincing excuse.

Whereas few parents would expect the lovers to remain physically aloof, some discretion is in order about overtly sexy forms of love-making in the public eye. Kisses, cuddles and fondling should be light and playful. Heavy intimacies that make onlookers feel spare deserve privacy.

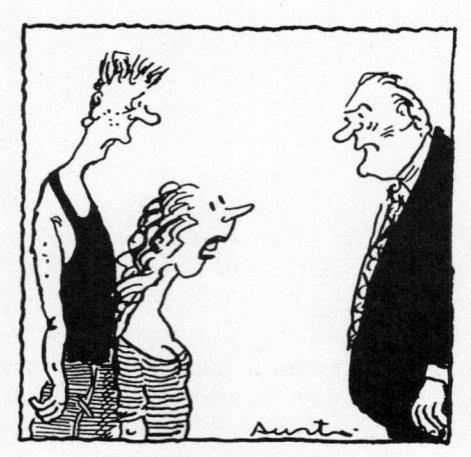

Bill is this month's long-term relationship, Daddy.

If the invitation is for an overnight stay and the couple are to share a bedroom for the first time under the parental roof, once again a sense of tact is likely to be appreciated. It is worth mentioning that this may have special relevance when the family member is a young daughter and her father may have long forgotten his own libidinous salad days.

If hospitality was offered by the hosts, a handwritten thank-you letter or card would probably come as a pleasant surprise.

Toy boy

Dark mutterings along the lines of 'He's too young for her' or 'She's too old for him' have sullied family discussions about matchmaking down the generations. It is hardly surprising, therefore, that not everyone feels comfortable with the Toy Boy syndrome.

The older woman who keeps company with a much younger male is a feature of our times. He may be a stud, a companion or the person's spouse – or all three. Sometimes he is little more than a 'walker', an escort who proverbially has no sexual interest in his date.

No matter, some adjustment of attitude is called for by those who take an ageist view of emotional entanglements – making due allowances for the law.

Older men have long enjoyed the favours of younger women; circumstances have come about in which older women now feel free to enjoy the favours of younger men.

Besides, the notion that a woman is bound to lose her sex appeal in maturity is almost daily confounded by the press as buzzy grandmothers sally forth on the arms of respectable, eligible younger males. As well, numerous albeit anonymous couples live to confirm the tale.

Age is always a sensitive subject and rarely more so than in this context. Very probably, both parties have been bored rigid by innuendo.

If courtesy is to be a guide, refraining from passing judgements in public based purely on the age differential of the couple is a golden rule. Similarly, the use in conversation of the sobriquet 'toy boy' in the company of the couple has to be tactfully eschewed. It could be said in mock irony but probably others present will be expected to forego the joke. It might also be thoughtful for older members to watch the number of times in conversation that a reference to the fact that the younger person 'Would be too young to remember' whatever historical event was being discussed, crops up.

Reverse age differentials may also have to be considered in an affair in which the man is of advanced years and his girlfriend a relative babe. Considerate friends are advised to be diplomatic about meting out the type of respectful behaviour which implies the recipient is an old buffer. Younger males might bite back the idea of addressing him formally as the member of an older generation, or of implying in any way that as a man he is past it.

Unavailable

Discouraging a male pest who won't take no for an answer takes persistence and tact in equal measures. It is certainly tricky if you do not wish to seem rude. And even when you are prepared to tell him straight, there is no

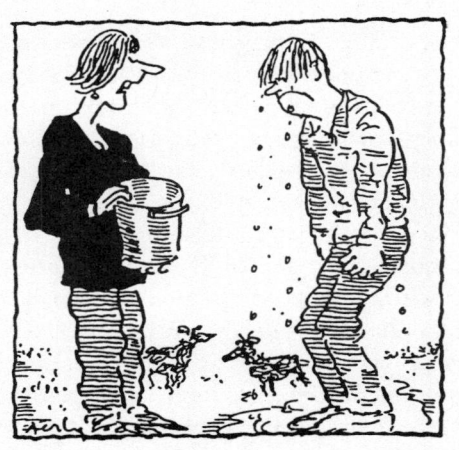

I'm sorry, but it always works with the dogs.

knowing whether this right-on form of rejection will not exacerbate the situation.

A rule which underlies all approaches is to avoid conveying any signals that could be misconstrued as encouragement – this bearing in mind that to a persistent follower, the merest half-smile or friendly conversational exchange may be taken as a come-on.

If a meeting is for some reason inescapable, better to agree to talk over lunch or a drink during the working week. The date offers a built-in excuse for a prompt getaway. It might be possible to ask if it would be all right if X or Y came too and made it a threesome.

If a face-to-face rejection seems crass, one gentler

approach is to take the person into your confidence and explain that you have met someone recently whom you have fallen for in a big way. Then again, mentioning a jealous partner, whether a fib or a fact, has its uses, but some independently-minded women might think they ought to manage this one under their own steam.

Sex counsellors usually advise against using abrasive language as a deterrent, or of taking actions which increase the feelings of powerlessness that may be felt by the rejected person. Insensitively handled, the situation can turn nasty.

If this should be the case and a nuisance becomes a threat, it is certainly unwise to laugh it off. Accepted guidelines in dealing with obsessive characters are to put as much distance as can be summoned between yourself and the pursuer. Try to avoid taking his telephone calls, don't reply to letters and return any presents sent. Adopt, as far as is practicable, erratic routines in going and coming.

Sometimes a reprisal can be a stream of unpleasant missives or scary messages left on the answering-machine. Not much can be done about the mail except to recognise the signs and refuse to open the letters but messages can be intercepted by an answering service, or by British Telecom. In extreme cases, it will be sensible to change a telephone number.

It is advisable to try to let friends or family know your whereabouts especially if you have changed your normal routine. If the person is a stalker and takes to hanging around the house, one practical measure is as much as possible to avoid being seen . At night, draw the curtains or blinds and an obvious move is to undress where you cannot be glimpsed from outside. Women living on their own are advised to alert friends or relations with a view to compiling an SOS telephone list.

In hard cases, the police should be informed with a full account of the incidents. Or it might be advisable to consult a solicitor on grounds of harassment.

The pest may well be female, in which case much of the above intelligence applies.

Kiss 'n' sell

The confidentiality of old love letters, and also of photographs, can pose a quandry.

When is it acceptable to allow outsiders to examine the private evidence of a romance? The question presses acutely in the instance — no longer as exceptional as at one time — of correspondence and mementos that have suddenly become hot property. When one of the lovers finds themselves thrust into the limelight, they may well come under pressure from the media to release the material.

Those who decide to kiss and tell may well discover

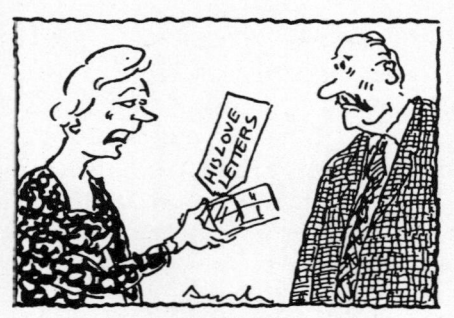

*They're photocopies. The originals
are with my publisher.*

that their motives will be questioned and found far from laudable. Jealousy or reprisal could have played a part in the decision to go public, reasons which may not remain hidden for long. The need to protect people on the periphery of the affair may deserve consideration. Living members of the family of the ex-lover, or any children of a parent in the case, might be specially vulnerable.

There can't be any doubt that it is discourteous, at the very least, to broadcast confidences entrusted to the recipient in good faith. Some would say unequivocally that the move is unethical. In real life though, the probability is that some balance will have to be found between loyalty and the temptation of monetary rewards.

Exceptions might be made for the sake of posterity and putting the record straight, in circumstances in which the correspondent might be shown to advantage, or, perhaps, when the affair happened a long time ago and the dust has long since settled.

Bedroom bliss

If just a smidgeon more thought was given to bedroomly habits as a subject apart, connubial contentment might have a longer run.

Sharing is the factor that may precipitate delight or disillusion. As countless newly-weds and couples cohabiting for the first time have discovered, the duality of occupying the heart of intimacy calls for more than a feisty sex life. Tact, tolerance and patience come into their own.

The notion of keeping up appearances in the bedroom may strike an unreal note as this is the one place where people want to be themselves. It is no bad thing though to arrest familiarity's slide into slobbery. There is an art to the state of undress for both sexes; it should be noted.

A bedroom more than any other room at home sparks differences of opinion on comfort, convenience and customs. What adds edge to the friction is that preferences are deeply held, often rooted in childhood, although on the surface the matter is superficial.

Tidiness tolerance varies enormously. Whereas one party may barely seem to notice that the place looks as if a wardrobe has exploded, others feel put out if a pair of pyjamas is folded awry. Order may be dismissed as anal retentive and fuddyduddy, disorder as thoughtless and time-wasting. Establishing a few must-dos or must-not-dos is at least a beginning. Finally, don't imbibe the other's glass of fresh water, do relegate the teddy bear to second place and try to be generous about moving over either way.

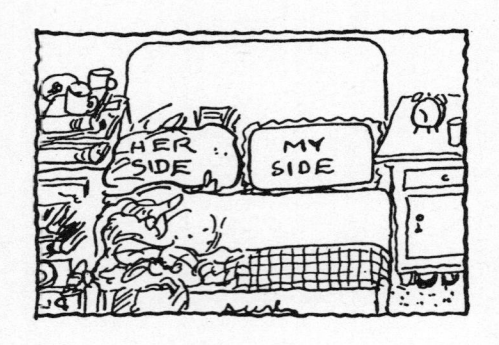

Two is company

Few need reminding that classic disturbers of connubial heaven are young children, and, it must be said, the house hound or cat. Each and all in their respective ways have a knack of turning up at exactly the wrong moment.

As the human animal likes to mate in private, a word must be put in for the partner who feels apprehensive

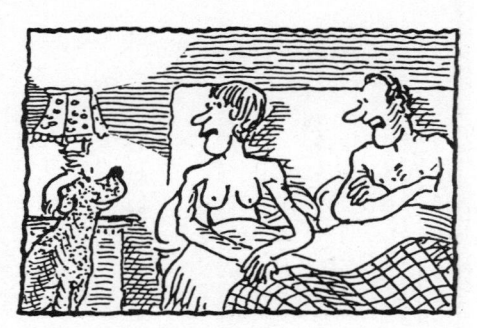

*If we must have that dog
in here, blindfold it.*

about making love when there is a chance of being intruded upon. Women, or so it is remarked, find the prospect of the imminent arrival of the patter of tiny feet, highly inhibiting. The one who has doubts does deserve consideration.

In any case, parenthood of tots and tinies generally heralds an abstemious phase of love-making in the interests of junior. Most parents live through this in a stoical manner, in the hopes of more promising nights ahead. All honour then to those who contrive to keep the flame of passion burning within the responsibilities of parenting.

As children grow, there is much to be said for inculcating the old-fashioned practice of knocking on a bedroom (or bathroom) door before entering. This custom has its uses, especially in households in which a parent is divorced or separated, and contemplates taking a new partner to bed. However, as with all family advice, much depends. What can be accomplished in surroundings with a contented young soul might well upset a dispirited or ailing member.

About house pets: once the pattern of sharing a bedroom with its owner has become routine, the habit is hard to break without protestation. If all attempts at reform fail and draconian measures are eschewed, there may be a case for taking a humorously relaxed view. After all, three can be company.

Betrayal

Cheating makes cowards of us all, to paraphrase the Bard. An eternal triangle – or infernal triangle as it has been described – plunges friends and acquaintances into a web of deception, game-playing, bluff and double-bluff.

What is primarily addressed here is just this point. How may those on the periphery of the affair best manage the diplomacy involved, especially if the wish exists to remain on friendly terms with more than one side?

Underlying the recommendations is a recognition that collusion is the best policy as a very general rule. To split on the gallivanter or philanderer is widely regarded as compounding the dirty tricks department. Tolerance of other's infidelity may show a lack of moral fibre, but it does at least give sinners the benefit of the doubt.

It is the small, day-to-day considerations that often represent the real posers. Many libidinous parties are members of the same social circle which may or may not create moments of potential awkwardness. Should a mutual friend invite both official and unofficial partner to the same party? The answer is depending. A small gathering seems to be tempting fate on the basis that there is nowhere for guests to escape to. On the other hand, an occasion with numbers, such as a wedding reception, a drinks party or reception, may offer a chance for the parties involved to keep their distance.

Risky, in the normal course of events, is the optimistic notion of inviting along a couple known to be in the throes of a contentious break-up. Emotional stress, allied to the bottle and the proximity of the inflammatory other, can easily over-topple normal restraints.

A more likely happening is espying the faithless one seated at a discreetly-placed restaurant table in the company of the new favourite. Vibes of guiltiness hover in the air. Practised observers who are uninvolved have learned to appear as if too wrapped up in their own concerns to notice the couple. If eye contact is made, a passing wave, or a friendly but carefully-abstracted nod should see the witness through.

The temptation to rubbish the culprit who seems to be the guilty party may well require second thoughts. In

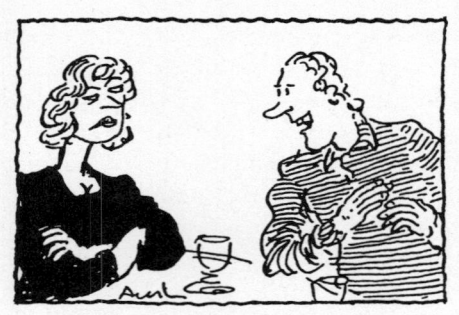

*My heart belongs to my wife,
but the rest of me is available.*

affairs of the heart, loyalties tend to change like the wind. Outspokenness may sound premature when the butt of your criticism is restored to favour. In short, staying neutral may be the path to continuing friendship.

Many and various are ways in which couples regulate the irregular. In some instances a mistress or boyfriend becomes a virtual institution within the family circle, thus avoiding messy marital split-ups. Close friends in such circumstances won't need any advice. But acquaintances might be forewarned that just because the liaison is recognised within the bosom of the family, this doesn't necessarily imply that it is an open subject for discussion or mention. As usual, watch-words are to avoid making the presumption of public knowledge.

Finally, is there any good advice that anyone has ever given someone in these circumstances that they haven't heard already or thought of themselves? Occasionally, as this account shows. One girlfriend of the wife of a pathologically philandering spouse was asked by the latter if she had any ideas on how she might deter him from bedding the au pair girls. As the result of this research the following took place. The wife duly found her husband with Hildegarde. 'Next time I find you in bed with my husband,' she said coolly, 'I'll make you spend the night with him.'

Afterthought

Good manners may have little to add to a bed of passion. Some do, others do not respond to mannerly forms of love-making; everyone to their own buzz.

Tactful behaviour and human understanding come into their own when sex just isn't all that good, or is a fiasco. Being sensitive to the situation can be a balm. Many a distraught lover can be restored to confidence through encouraging utterances as well as loving physical demonstrations of affection and acceptance.

Few will need to be reminded that recriminations are deadly in the circumstances. To say that someone has failed as a lover remains one of the unforgivable jibes, even in this age of brutal candour.

If the party hopes to continue in a sexual relationship,

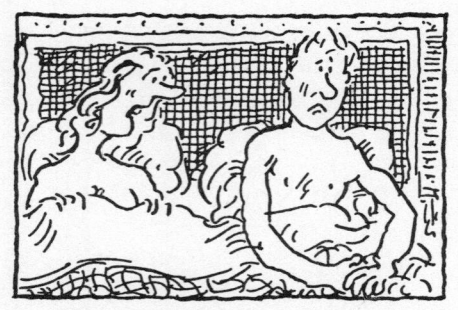

Never mind, you'll probably laugh about it tomorrow. I know I will.

a more subtle approach is needed. In place of silence or slumber some responses can be recommended. Whereas ecstasy is a fixed star, without a doubt, much encouragement may be found in degrees of comparative success that are part of any lesser experience.

The fun and satisfaction of closeness, physical intimacy in embracing or caressing and kissing, in being able to give the other person pleasure even if the stars did not rocket, are not to be kept to yourself alone.

The question of whether the one who feels they have disappointed should apologise in so many words, is probably governed as much by character as by any formal prompting. The gesture can be a simple way of putting things right or even of gallantly accepting responsibility, whether justified or no. Once again, a matter-of-fact delivery can be off-putting and can make the recipient feel as if they were a toe that has been trodden on my mistake.

Kiss and try again is the most promising response.

'Bye

A wit once remarked that he thought it rude to go to bed with someone just once. That is as maybe, but the reflection does call into question acceptable ways of parting after a momentary indulgence or one-night stand.

It would be sad to think that the ultimate physical intimacy did not merit some gesture of appreciation. Even a verbal expression of thanks would be better than nothing. Abrupt endings are usually hurtful when they occur despite a mutual understanding that only a limited engagement was on the cards.

The defecting partner may say something along the lines of 'I'll speak to you soon', which would leave the matter of any further commitment open-ended. Obviously, if the experience was sensational, yet tricky circumstances mean this has to be the end of the affair, expressing delight in the memory and sadness in parting goes without saying.

As is mentioned elsewhere in this little guide, the one unforgivable insult is to state that your partner is no good in bed, and that includes whatever euphemism is employed meaning the same thing.

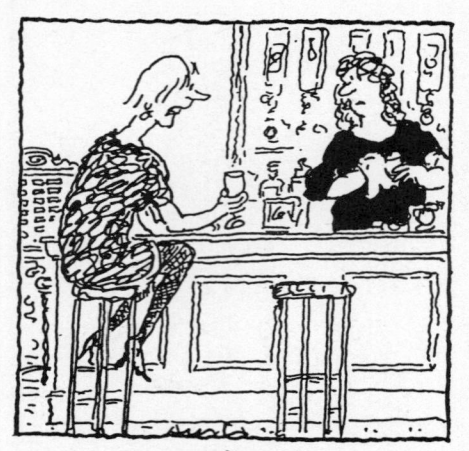

I knew it was over when he did 'Just one of those things' on karaoke night.

No go

A male lament. Not tonight, because she:
- has to get up at dawn
- has a cold coming on
- must get to the end of the chapter
- couldn't miss the final reel of the movie
- has a funny discharge
- has awful backache
- is just about to zzizz off
- has a heavy period

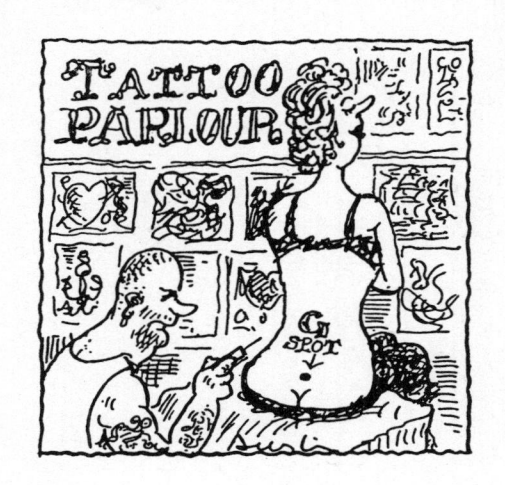

- thinks her spots are infectious
- has taken a Valium
- absolutely must finish her work
- forgot to bring anything
- is sure the children will barge in
- has to call Mum last thing
- is in the middle of a wonderful dream
- has overdone the sun worship
- has a throbbing headache
- has strained a muscle when working out
- is completely OUT, dead, collapsed
- will be herself in the morning

All the excuses above have been worn thin by women who want to cry off the advances of their mate. The best that can be said about the euphemisms is that at least these show an unwillingness to offend. It is axiomatic that the male should use his second sense about knowing when and when not to take no for an answer. It can be an affront when the signals are misread, and men use their strength to insist.

Having said that, this seems the place to note that sex is the best sleeping pill, energizer, and when things go well, puts lovers in an optimistic frame of mind. Just a thought before the moment of rebuff.